THE WAR AGAINST CANCER

FOODS YOU SHOULD AVOID

TO BEAT CANCER

SIENNA SILVERTON

Copyright ©2018 by Inspired Word Publishers. All rights reserved.

Printed in the United States of America

No part of this book may be reproduced in any written, electronic, recording, or photocopying without written permission of the publisher or author.

ISBN-13: 978-1726490412

ISBN-10: 1726490416

Why I Wrote This Book

Cancer is a global health concern which is almost at the threshold of being a health crisis. Incidences of cancer are on the rise, even places which previously did not have to worry about cancer are now faced with it.

Here are some statistics about cancer from the World Health Organization website:

"Cancer is the second leading cause of death globally and was responsible for 8.8 million deaths in 2015. Globally, nearly 1 in 6 deaths is due to cancer."

"Approximately 70% of deaths from cancer occur in low- and middle-income countries."

According to A Cancer Journal for Clinicians, *"In 2018, 1,735,350 new cancer cases and 609,640 cancer deaths are projected to occur in the United States."*

These figures should get us concerned. Too many people are dying from cancer unnecessarily. We and our loved ones do not have to become the next victim of cancer. We need to have the information to help us prevent, manage, and treat cancer.

The most important thing, however, is to know what causes cancer and do all that is necessary to reduce the incidences of cancer. This book is my part to win the war against cancer.

Why You Should Read This Book

This book is invaluable for anyone who wants to know ***how to deal with cancer or those who want to prevent it all together, by effectively managing diet*** for cancer prevention.

More than that, this book questions the commitment to curing cancer by raising questions about ***why cancer cannot be cured despite the billions of dollars that have been channeled into its research and treatment***.

This book explores why cancer is increasing and looks into the various risk factors. It discusses ***why your location could be the difference between developing cancer and not having cancer***, and why cancer is all about what you eat. ***Why the food we eat makes all the difference when it comes to cancer***.

Learn more about the risky foods you need to avoid, the costs of treating cancer for those with insurance and those without, as well as the 'elephant in the room' in cancer research circles, ***whether cancer treatment is now a business and there is no real urgency to get a cure***.

What you will read here will help you make the right decisions to prevent cancer by eating the right foods, those who are already dealing with cancer will ***get insights into the treatment options available and the cost factors involved***.

I hope you find this life-saving information valuable.

Table Of Contents

Chapter 1. Losing the War Against Cancer 2
    The Rate of Cancer Is Increasing 3
    The Countries Most At Risk 5
    The Demographics of Cancer 6
    Why Does Cancer Treatment Fail? 7

Chapter 2. The Economics of Cancer 16
    Cost Of Cancer On The Rise 16
    Total Cost of Cancer Treatment 18
    Hidden Cost During Cancer Treatment 20
    The Cost Of Treatment With Insurance 21
    The Cost of Treatment Without Insurance 22
    The Business of Cancer 22

Chapter 3. Location Matters 30
    Poor Countries Eat Better 31
    Rich Countries Eat Poorer 36

Chapter 4. It's The Food 38
    Foods That Increase Cancer Risk 38
    Foods That Lower Cancer Risk 41
    Dietary Weight Control 42

Chapter 5. The Diet That Causes Cancer 44
    Foods That Cause Cancer 44
    Drinks That Cause Cancer 53

Chapter 1

Losing the War Against Cancer

Cancer is one of the foremost killer diseases found in the world today. With so many people being diagnosed and its high mortality rate, it is a health problem that is giving researchers sleepless nights and causing a financial burden on families and the health sector. It seems we are losing the war against cancer.

Cancer is a medical term that is used to describe the abnormal and uncontrollable growth of one or more cells in parts of the body causing tumors or buildup of unhealthy cells in these parts of the body.

There are so many types of cancer, actually over 200 types, but they can be divided into categories by stages, severity and the cells that have been affected. These main types are;

- **Carcinomas**

Carcinomas are cancers that affect epithelial cells usually found on the skin and are also present in the tissues surrounding and protecting internal organs e.g. breast cancers, lung cancers among others.

- **Leukemia**

Leukemia is a type of cancer that affects the blood when too many white blood cells are produced, uncontrollably, by the bone marrow.

- **Sarcomas**

Sarcoma is a type of cancer that affects bones and soft tissues like tendons.

- **Lymphatic System Cancer**

Lymphatic system cancer is a type of cancer that affects the lymphatic system, which is responsible for carrying white blood cells from the lymph nodes, located in different parts of the body, to the rest of the body to fight off germs and diseases.

- **Brain and Spinal Cord Cancer**

Brain and spinal cord cancer affect the brain and the spinal cord in the human body. It is mostly characterized by headaches, loss of vision or loss of balance.

You are more at risk to develop cancer due to certain lifestyle behaviors or your genetic make-up. Once you understand the risk factors that might increase your chances of developing cancer, it can help you avoid the catalysts or decide which cancer screening test to take so that you can get ahead of it before it develops.

The Rate of Cancer Is Increasing

The rate of cancer has been increasing over the years, but this is not to say that progress isn't being made in the fight against it. According to the findings of a report done in by Professor Peter Sasieni (Sasieni), cancer reports were 1 in 3, but that rate has increased to 1 in 2. This drastic change makes one question why the rate is increasing.

Why are people more prone to developing this disease now than in the past?

There has been a lot of advancements in medicine and technology that prolong human life. According to Prof. Sasieni's report done in the UK, more than three – quarters of cancer patients are people over the age of 60 years old. The reason behind people being diagnosed with this disease when they get older is because cancer is a disease of the genes. (Sasieni)

Genes are the genetic code (DNA) that holds instructions for the workings of our cells in the body. As more time passes, mistakes tend to accumulate in this code causing complications in the growth of new cells. Scientists have been able to identify these mistakes, through the advanced medical technology, and how these mistakes kick-start their journey to become cancerous cells in the human body.

This is not to say that there is nothing we can do to avoid these mistakes in our genetic make-up. The way one lives his or her life will greatly determine if these errors can be slowed down or sped up, leaving them to decide how they want to live their lives and how much they want to improve their quality of life. Lifestyle, genetics, family history, exposure to viruses, jobs done or the air that is breathed are some of the things that can determine if they will develop cancer or not.

'Lifetime risk' is a simple but complex concept to wrap one's head around. The likelihood of a child developing cancer at any point in their life will greatly depend on assumptions about the cancer risk in the future rather than today. This is done by estimating incidence rates in the past and determination of how likely the child is to develop it in the future. Although this method is effective, it's limited in the sense that incidences are not likely to stay the same throughout their lives.

Professor Sasieni and his team, whose report is published in the *British Journal of Cancer*, the year a person is born will be compared to the year when the child reaches 60 years. The estimate is done by looking at past incidences and coming up with a risk rate for the child's future chance of developing cancer when they reach 60 years.

This research showed that someone born in 1930 has a risk rate of 1 in 3 but by the time they get to sixty years old, this figure will have risen to 1 in 2. This means that as time progresses, the risk of acquiring cancer increases and an individual becomes more prone to developing it.

THE COUNTRIES MOST AT RISK

According to researchers at the University of Washington, for cancer incidences between 1990 and 2016, cancer incidences had risen to 28 percent, which is approximately 17.2 million people in the world. Together with these findings, they also revealed some of the countries with the highest incidences of new cancer cases compared to other countries in the world.

Topping the list is Australia with 743.8 per 100,000 people. New Zealand follows by having 524.8 per 100,000 people and the United States with 532.9 per 100,000 people. As much as these countries rank highest on the list, there are also countries that have the lowest rates of reported cases of cancer.

Syria tops the list by having 85 per 100,000 people, followed by Bhutan, a small country that borders India, with 86 patients out of 100,000, and Algeria in Africa with 86.7 patients per 100,000 people. (Death Express UK, n.d.) The research also pointed out that developed countries have a higher rate of cancer diagnosis than in developing countries. This is because these countries have such advanced technologies that use a lot of energy causing cancer development risk to be higher. (Express, n.d.)

THE DEMOGRAPHICS OF CANCER
Cancer is the leading cause of disease with an estimated 14.1 million cases in 2012. The number varies between men having a percentage of 53%, estimating to about 7.4 million people being diagnosed, and women with 47%, estimating to about 6.7 million people. (The world age Standardised Incidence rate, n.d.)

If considering the estimates for males and females in different countries, France has the highest incidences in males with 385 incidences per 100,000 people. Denmark, on the other hand, has the highest female cancer rates with 329 incidences per 100,000. (Ferlay J, 2012)

There are four common types of cancers that occur worldwide. Lung cancer was the most common cancer worldwide in men, occurring in more than 1 in 10 of all the cancers that are diagnosed in men. This is because men are the highest users of tobacco than women thus the high rate.

Breast cancer has also been one of the highest diagnosed cancers in women than in men. This is because women have a higher risk of developing breast cancer due to the formation of mammary glands that develop during childbirth and breastfeeding.

African countries do not have such a high rate of cancer development with only 85 incidences in 100,000 people. Algeria reports the fewest incidences of cancer than other African countries. Syria, with only 86 per 100,000 people, is also counted as one of the countries with the least cases of cancer incidences in the world.

Including both sexes, lung, breast, and colorectal cancer is the leading cause of cancer incidences in the world. (Ferlay J, 2012)

WHY DOES CANCER TREATMENT FAIL?

Today, there are many cancer treatments available, but certain factors should be considered when choosing which type of treatment to accept. These factors are; the type of cancer, the stage of cancer, that is, how much it has grown and how far it has spread, the age of the patient, the overall health of the patient and, other health problems of the patient. Here are some of the various forms of cancer treatments that exist today:

Surgery is a procedure whereby the surgeon removes cancer growth from your body and it is also used to find out how far cancer has spread. This method has been used to treat cancer for many years and it has proved very effective since it has very good outcomes.

Radiation Therapy can be described as a cancer treatment where high doses of radiation such as x-rays, electron beams, protons or high energy particles are used to kill cancer cells and to also shrink cancer tumors. It works by making small breaks in the genetic make-up (DNA) inside cells making them stop growing, dividing and eventually dying.

Chemotherapy is the treatment of cancer by use of drugs to kill cancer cells and to also control the growth of these cells. It has an advantage over surgery and radiation because it works throughout the body when eliminating cancer cells in the body. This method aims to cure, control and palliation cancer cells from the body thus giving the body a chance to fight these cancer cells.

The other forms of treatment are Immunotherapy, which is a cancer treatment that usually helps the immune system to fight cancer, and targeted therapy, which is a cancer treatment method that targets changes in the cancer cells that help them spread, grow and divide in the human body. This gives the body a fighting chance when it comes to eliminating the cancer cells and controlling their growths.

Although these treatment methods are effective when it comes to treating cancer, the survival rates of these treatments are usually very low. Survival rates describe the portion of people having the same type of cancer and at the same stage will live up to a certain time after being diagnosed. This is not to say that they will tell you how long you will have to live, but it will give you a better idea and understanding of how likely the treatment will be successful and for how long.

Five-year survival rates are the statistics that most cancer diagnosis is given. It describes the percentage of people who have a good chance of living at least 5 years after the cancer diagnosis. These relative survival rates are the most accurate ways of estimating the best chance a cancer patient has to survive. They normally compare cancer patients with similar diagnosis in the overall population.

As much as survival rates are best at predicting the estimates, they largely depend on outcomes of a large number of people who had the disease in the past, but they are not accurate at predicting what will happen to that particular person's case. Another limitation of this statistic is that it is based on when the cancer is first diagnosed but does not apply to when the cancer spreads or cancers that come back later.

An example of a cancer survival rate report is the stomach cancer survival rates. According to a report by the National Cancer Database for people with stomach cancer and have been treated with surgery between 2004 and 2008, their survival rates reduced from 2004 to 2008. It is also important to note that with this research, the survival rates did not also put in an account that people with the stomach cancer can die from other things other than cancer (Database, 2017).

According to Katie Forster, a health correspondent for the independent online, 'Patients with the six deadliest cancers, that is, Pancreatic cancer, Liver, brain, lung, esophageal and stomach cancer, have the least survival rates compared to all other types of cancers.' These people are less likely to survive for the five-year survival rates thus getting the name 'silent killer.'

As much as cancer treatments have a lot of upsides to the control of cancer cells in the body, there are quite a number of ways that these treatments can poison one's body and leave it more damaged than when they started using these treatments. We will look at two treatments that have proved fatal in terms of poisoning one's body, and these treatments are; Radiation therapy and Chemotherapy.

Radiation therapy, as we have seen, uses high energy beams to treat cancer. But like any other drugs, they have quite a number of side effects that have proved poisonous to the human body. When radiation therapy is used, the high energy frequency not only destroys the cancer cells, but it also affects and damages healthy cells and tissues that are near the treatment area and treatment tissues of the body being affected.

These radiation side effects reactions start during the second or third week of treatment. The side effects can even last weeks after the final treatment has been given and this makes it hard to cope.

Some of the side effects of radiation treatment are:

Hair loss; if the place being treated for cancer is aimed at the part of the body that grows hair e.g. the scalp. Another side effect of this therapy is **skin problems-** skin dryness, itching, blistering or peeling are some of the effects on skin exposed to radiation depending on the area the radiation treatment is being exposed to. These skin problems usually go away a few weeks after the final treatment.

Feeling fatigued is one of the most frustrating side effects of this treatment. The feeling of being exhausted all the time will also depend on whether you are receiving other cancer treatments, but the general feeling of fatigue is related to all the cancer treatments available.

As much as the above side effects are short-term, radiation can cause some other long-term effects that develop long after the final treatment is administered. With radiation therapy, the **risk of later developing another cancer** is high because the white blood cells that are used to fight these cancerous cells are also destroyed during the treatment.

Other side effects of radiation are; **dry mouth, sore gums,** having **difficulty when swallowing, nausea, lymphedema** (a type of swelling), **stiffness in the jaw** area of the mouth, **tooth decay, chest pains** and **difficulty breathing,** shortness of breath, **breast and nipple soreness,** and **shoulder stiffness. Radiation pneumonia** can also occur between 2 to 6 weeks after the radiation therapy is started.

Chemotherapy treatment is where drugs are used in treating cancer cells and controlling their growth. It is also a very effective method of controlling cancer but the side effects can leave your body weaker than before you started the treatment.

Some of the side effects associated with chemotherapy treatments are:

Nausea and vomiting. Because of the high dose and powerful properties of chemotherapy, once ingested as tablets or as intravenous injection, chemotherapy can mess with the body's hormones and thus cause one to feel nauseated and sometimes even vomit.

Diarrhea is also another side effect of chemotherapy especially when tablets are used. The doctor can prescribe drugs to deal with this side effect but they usually last as long as one is under this treatment. This side effect can affect your diet and will make you feel uncomfortable throughout the treatment.

Other side effects from chemotherapy include **rectal bleeding, incontinence, bladder irritation**, acquiring other **opportunistic infections** since the body defense mechanism is lowered, **hormonal changes, headaches, loss of energy, sleepiness, having sleep disorders** among other side effects.

There are other side effects that affect only men and women when they are receiving cancer treatments.

Men can experience **sexual problems** e.g. erectile dysfunction (inability to get or maintain an erection when sexually active), they may also experience **lowered sperm count** and also **reduced sperm activity**.

For women, these treatments can cause an array of effects. Provided are just a few of these side effects. **Changes in menstruation** and also **stoppage of menstruation** can be experienced during these treatments. A woman can also experience **symptoms of menopause such as vaginal itching, burning, and dryness. Infertility issues** (inability to conceive a child or to maintain a pregnancy to full term) are also experienced.

Everyone experiences cancer treatments side effects differently, and every person gets different symptoms from the treatments. Due to this, doctors will also prescribe other drugs to cope with these side effects and this will cause even further reactions in the body rather than the effects from the cancer treatments.

It is vital to understand the treatment the doctor prescribes. With this knowledge, you can make more informed decisions on which treatment to use. This way, you can minimize the damage that these treatments may have on your body.

Chapter Summary

In this chapter, we have defined what cancer is, explored the major types of cancer that exist, and the factors that might increase the chance of developing cancer during one's life.

There are also various statistics that show which countries are most affected by certain types of cancer giving one an idea of how the cancer pandemic has affected the world and different states. The survival rates and how they are calculated are important because they give one an idea of how likely they are to survive a cancer diagnosis.

As much as there are various treatments that can be used to cure and control cancer cells in the body, there also exists severe side effects that these treatments can cause to the human body. These treatments can poison the body and thus cause other harmful effects than before the treatment was given.

Chapter 2

The Economics of Cancer

One would expect that due to the advancement in the treatment and research of cancer, the financial burden imposed on patients would have reduced dramatically. Curiously, the opposite is true!

The costs of cancer treatment have been rising steadily over the years. Cancer treatment is financially burdensome and the medical bills keep on piling up as more treatment sessions are needed to control the growth of cancer cells in the body.

Additionally, there are extra expenses which elevate the cost of cancer treatment such as travel and lodging expenses in cases where there is no local access to the necessary specialists in the area.

Some people have questioned this trend, especially, in the wake of studies and research that predict a further increase in the costs to treat cancer. It has been called the 'business of cancer' thus the need to understand the economics of cancer.

How exactly has cancer treatment increased over the years?

Cost Of Cancer On The Rise

The cost of health care has been rising over the years; developed countries like the US have increased their health care spending over the years. According to a report given by a US government health agent on Washington Reuters, the rise of prices for medical goods and services will make the US Health spending rise to 5.3 percent in 2018 compared to a 2017 estimate of 4.6 percent.

There are primary drivers that are contributing to such an increase in health care spending. These include:

- **An aging population,**

- **Increasing enrollment of the aging population to the health care system,**

- **The rise of medical goods and services prices** and lastly,

- **An increase in disposable income from the people living in the United States.**

Due to expected growth and an aging population, the aggregate financial burden of cancer treatment in the US will increase significantly. The modern treatment and screening technology available today enable patients to receive a world-class medical diagnosis. As much as this technology is available, the cost of medical care is expected to rise due to these technological advancements.

Increase in aspects like health care expenditures, productivity loss and the morbidity for patients and families affected by this disease are some of the expenditures that cancer patients will have to go through.

Monetary valuation of resources that are used in the treatment of cancer and the loss of opportunities caused by cancer are all measured as costs when estimating the economic burden of cancer. Considering a cost estimate for a period e.g. 2001-2002, the estimate will include patients that are diagnosed within this period for the overall cancer estimate cost.

According to a study published by Dr. Springer Berlin Heidelberg, once the cancer drugs go on the market, the prices increase over time even when faced with competition. (Heidelberg). This study was done with an aim of looking at the relationship of cancer drugs with forces in the market that influence price changes.

TOTAL COST OF CANCER TREATMENT

Cancer treatment results in opportunities and economic loss for the patients, families, employers and the overall society at large. Losses like financial loss, morbidity, reduced quality of life and premature death are all measured as costs when estimating the economic burden of cancer.

The costs can be distributed among various periods of the disease i.e., initial care, recurrence, and end of life care. Cancer treatment costs have two domains where cancer costs can be estimated from:

1. **Direct medical costs**: these are those costs associated with the direct services that the

patients receive. Such costs include hospitalizations, physician visits, surgery, radiation therapy, chemotherapy, and immunotherapy.

2. **Indirect Costs:** These are monetary costs which are associated with the amount of time spent in receiving medical care by the patients, the time lost from work and other activities that the patient is involved in and the loss of the productivity of the patient due to premature death.

So, what are the factors that contribute to the rising costs of cancer treatment?

One factor that greatly contributes to this rise in cost is that **cancer treatment is needed urgently**. Cancer patients and caretakers usually act immediately, unlike with diabetes which can be regulated overtime with a proper diet. Cancer can kill a victim within months which can be painful and debilitating. Thus, cancer prompts the victims and their families to use costly procedures such as chemotherapy and radiation treatment to cure and control it.

Health insurance has helped a lot of people manage the costs of cancer treatment. Unfortunately, there are many that are not insured, making a few cancer victims dig deep into their pockets for treatment. Tragically, sometimes insurance companies decide not to pay for treatments if the medical costs are too high leaving the patient with little chance for survival.

Hidden Cost During Cancer Treatment

Cancer is a very expensive disease. Not only will one consider medical and drugs costs, but there are also other costs associated with the treatment. These costs are unforeseen and usually add up very quickly in the course of the treatment. Some of these costs are:

Travel Expenses: These are costs involved in getting to and from treatment. If the cancer treatment center is far from where the patient lives, the patient will have to incur transportation costs to reach the treatment center.

Patients along with the families or caregivers living with them usually see an increase in the **cost of living**. Since the cancer patient will usually be at home while they fight this disease, the electricity bill can go up, the cost of food also increases and also the payment of additional supplements that will enable the patient to recuperate.

The house also needs to be cleaned. The patient will not have the energy to clean and the caregiver may not have the time to clean the house and look after the patient. One will have to find a paid housekeeper who will clean the house and wash clothes.

The treatment of cancer can be disabling and time-consuming for both the patient and the caregiver. When the patient **loses income** that would have helped them during their recovery, it can cause a great deal of frustration.

The Cost Of Treatment With Insurance

Insurance has been around for decades giving people peace of mind when it comes to handling certain risks that can occur in a person's life, like cancer. Medical insurance is a health plan that helps pay for medical treatments.

Some of the insurance rights that patients have when a cancer risk has occurred are: **there can be no cancellation of the insurance due to cancer developing, the insurance cannot deny one cover in case they develop cancer**, and finally, the **coverage includes children who develop cancer**. The patient is therefore protected against a cancer risk developing, thus, reducing the financial stress that the patient might have.

Although the medical coverage from the insurance company cannot completely cover the cost of treatment, it does help in a huge way, compared to having to handle the entire financial burden out of pocket.

There can be some limitations to the insurance cover on the treatment costs though. It is important for you to consult with the insurance company about these limitations so that you are informed on the full scope of cancer treatment coverage provided by the insurance company.

The Cost of Treatment Without Insurance

We have already established that cancer treatments are very expensive. Although many hospitals have increased the amount of charity care offered to patients needing cancer treatment, there is a limit to how much time they can devote to uninsured patients without payment.

Government health care plans have greatly helped patients who are uninsured because the costs are just too high for them to manage on their own, thus posing a threat to their health. In the US, the government has a Medicaid plan where, if these patients apply, they can start treatment and they usually take 3 to 6 months for the cover to be approved, compared to private insurance companies which have a waiting period of 12 months for the cover to be approved.

Regrettably, it has been proven that uninsured patients are usually charged 43 times more than the insured. A study by the students from the University of North Carolina at Chapel Hill, reported in the Carolina Breast Study report in 2013, showed that patients diagnosed with breast cancer and have no insurance cover, most likely, end up being charged more than their insured counterparts. (Carolina)

The Business of Cancer

"It is true to say that cancer treatment is a multi-billion dollar industry due to the high cost of treatment available today," says Dr. Julian Whitaker, M.D, founder of Whitaker Wellness Institute. He further asked, "Why are people terrified when they hear the word cancer?

Because they know it [conventional cancer treatment] doesn't work."

The point he is making here is that the cancer 'industry' makes too much money from money donated for research to risk finding or announcing a cure. The financial incentive is in the research of cancer and finding a cure would interrupt the stream of money flowing into this 'industry'.

Treating cancer makes more money than if a cure for cancer is found. Billions of dollars have been put into research that has not yielded any concrete results from time immemorial. Instead of resulting in a cure for cancer, this money has gone to fund the discovery of even more expensive cancer treatments that cause more harm rather than good to the human body.

The cure for cancer would mean that the money put into research would dry up, thus, if the cancer researchers want a continuing flow of money, then it is in their best interest not to find a cure. Money is the main reason why a cure for cancer has never been found. This is a very sad reality and reflection of the kind of world we live in.

Alternative cancer treatments that could actually cure cancer are considered wishful thinking or hocus pocus because it actually threatens the bottom line of mainstream cancer treatment. Cancer patients are seen as dollar signs to these researchers because their aim is not to save lives but to continue earning more money.

Why do you think up until now, in this advanced world of technology, cancer has no cure despite being diagnosed so much earlier than in the past? Why do you think that the more people that use these conventional cancer treatments like chemotherapy and radiation, the more their lifespan tends to decrease compared to when they would not have used these treatments?

The truth is, the so-called cancer treatments do not really cure cancer. Most patients are never really cured and those who are treated will always have a recurrence of the disease and die from it. Consequently, the cynics and skeptics have always raised the possibility that the lack of a cure is deliberate, especially considering all the money being poured into cancer drugs and treatment research.

People are actually poisoning their bodies in contrast to how they may have coped without these treatments. The treatments are even responsible for causing further spread of the cancer cells in other parts of the body, where they were not before.

Dr. Thomas N. Seyfried, Ph.D. a known researcher in Genetics and Biochemistry did a study on cancer as a metabolic disease and the following are some of his findings on the research:

- There has been no real progress made in managing advanced or metastatic cancer for more than 40 years. The number of people who have died from cancer each year has changed a little in more than 10 years.

- Many cancers are discovered after they have metastasized and have already spread to other locations in the human body.

- There is a common mechanism for treating all cancers since they are not really different in metamorphosis.

- Cancer has a genetic origin but other factors such as toxic exposure like radiation and chemotherapy create conditions where these cancer cells can develop.

- Genetic abnormalities cause cancer but they are a consequence of cancer and not the cause of it.

- Cancer is viewed as a genetic disease but this is no longer credible.

- The cancer cells largely depend on glucose and glutamine metabolism for survival, growth, and proliferation.

- If one restricts glucose and glutamine, it can compromise cancer cell growth and survival.

- Antioxidants largely prevent and reduce the risk of cancer in a person.

- Lifestyle changes and food should be managed so as to prevent cancer.

- Once cancer becomes recognized as a metabolic disease, cancer management and prevention will emerge.

What Dr. Seyfried was saying is, the cure for cancer is to starve cancer cells so that they die, while feeding the rest of the body so that it grows stronger and use its natural immune system to resist cancer. A high fat, low carbohydrate diet should be employed if anyone is to have a chance of winning this war against cancer. (Dr. Thomas N. Seyfried, 2012)

Dr. Gonzales, the developer of pancreatic enzyme therapy, made this statement during an interview with the National Cancer Institute, "War on cancer has been a failure due to a combination of politics, money, greed, and corruption in the world." He understood that there is no way humans can win this war against cancer by the conventional treatments that doctors are prescribing.

Carbohydrate has become a deadly food group that most people seem to be victimized by. Carbohydrate has been proven to cause diabetes, heart disease, Alzheimer's, and cancer. A breakfast that consists of carbohydrate is really dangerous but that is what is being advised on our televisions to eat more of.

Today, there are more carbohydrate addicts than in the past, and that is why diseases like cancer are more on the rise today than in the past. People, without knowing, keep feeding their cancer with carbohydrate and the cancer cells keep on growing despite the chemo, radiation, and surgery. They have refused the idea that carbs have anything to do with their condition.

The only way to be free from all this brainwash is to know that your body has its own defense mechanism. It has an immune system that when it is treated right, then, any disease that may come can be dealt with. People have been brainwashed to believe that doctors are our saviors, and we should trust their every word.

People have given doctors so much power that they do not realize it when they are steered in the wrong direction. The drugs that are administered to most patients are only making the situation worse instead of making it better.

People should realize that the slogan "An apple a day, keeps the doctor away" is true to the letter. Changing one's lifestyle by eating healthy and exercising are the only ways that people can keep their bodies healthy and strong. Make a change today and start living a healthy life.

If you have a headache, you do not have to go to a doctor for medicine. There are other nonmedicinal things that you can do to relieve your headache. The medicine the doctor is going to give you will have other side effects which are more harmful than the headache.

The medicine also lowers your immune system, making your body dependent on the drugs. If you can just decide to live healthily, then a world without cancer can be achieved. Make that change today, and start living healthy, and you will see the difference.

CHAPTER SUMMARY

Cancer is a deadly disease that has been increasing over the past few years. More people are being diagnosed with cancer than in the past. The future will be very scary if things continue as they are. From estimates of 1 in 3 to 1 in 2, cancer has become increasingly scary because it means that more people are going to develop it in the future.

With this increase, there have been advancements in cancer treatment and this has given a lot of people hope of surviving this pandemic. But their hopes are sometimes short-lived because for one to access such treatments, they have to have fortunes to be able to keep up with the treatments.

Cancer treatments are very expensive and sometimes insurance companies can help cover these costs. They have been a beacon of hope for people diagnosed with cancer. However, as much as insurance has helped more people to receive treatment, they are often limited to how much cover they can give. Patients do have rights on the cover, but you will find that insurance companies have found ways to limit these covers, leaving patients stranded.

Curiously, research to find a cure for cancer has been going on for decades, but the results have proven futile. Have researchers become greedy and could a cure put a stop to their cash flow? Researchers continue to come up with more expensive cancer treatments that drain patients' pockets and later on, they die after spending all their life savings on 'treatment'.

People like Dr. Syfried have done a lot in terms of finding a solution in all this confusion. His report on the study of cancer suggests that a good change of lifestyle and the food that one eats can greatly minimize the effects of cancer in patients today. His findings have been a milestone in the war against cancer and have helped a lot of people combat the disease.

With alternative treatments and lifestyle changes, people have a chance against cancer and they can now hope that a true solution to this problem has been found.

One question remains. Will people be bold enough to take control of their life and not leave it in the hands of the ineffective yet financially profitable cancer treatment machine?

Chapter 3

Location Matters

Being healthy is such a wide concept that many people do not understand what it actually means. Most people think that being healthy only involves sweating off the calories ingested but it is so much more than that.

There are various components that make up good health in someone's life but the leading components of a healthy life are summed up in two types of environments. The first environment is the external environment; this is an environment where people have access to health information, hospitals, doctors, drugs, surgeons, and caregivers to manage their health.

The other type of environment, which comes as a challenge for many, is the internal environment. Factors like personal diet and exercise are considered in this environment. This is the most important of all the environments because it prevents a lot of health issues that might result in someone needing to visit a hospital for treatment.

As strange as it may seem, it is a fact that people in third world countries are generally much healthier than people in developed countries. As much as developed countries have the best external environment when it comes to being healthy, their internal environment suffers gruesomely because they have not maintained a culture of eating healthy foods. Accordingly, **when it comes to cancer risk, your location matters**.

POOR COUNTRIES EAT BETTER

The main reason why third world countries eat healthier than developed countries is that people in the third world countries do not have enough money to buy damaging processed foods that are often purchased in the developed world. People in poor countries have broadly stuck to healthy natural diets which are mainly fed by subsistence farming.

Simply put, people in poor countries grow what they eat. They do not buy processed food which has been depleted of the primary nutrients and are sold in the refined form. Poor countries, largely by economic circumstance, have to eat natural foods which are far less expensive.

People in developed countries have a problem when it comes to calorie intake because many of them have bought into the lie that all calories are the same. They do not understand that calories are just a measure of how much energy is provided in the food but it does not inform about the energy level that food gives to a person.

Dr. Fumiaki Imamura from the University of Cambridge conducted research where an analysis of healthy food intake like fruits, vegetables, legumes, whole grains, fish, food containing fiber and foods containing omega 3 was done. He compared this analysis to the consumption of unhealthy foods like sugary drinks, saturated fats, sodium and processed meats and came up with the following report.

Sub Saharan African countries, especially West Africa, who consumed the healthy foods, ranked better than wealthier regions in North America and Europe, who mostly consumed the unhealthy foods. Dr. Imamura concluded that most developed countries around the world have bad eating habits and it is only getting worse by the day.

The study found that as much as worldwide consumption of healthy foods have greatly increased, high-income countries have also increased their unhealthy food intake which contributes to the rise in non-communicable diseases like cancer, respiratory illness, cardiovascular disease and also the increase of immature death rates in these countries.

Dr. Fumiaki Imamura stated, "By 2020, projections indicate that non- communicable diseases like cancer will account for 75 percent of all deaths around the world. When people start to improve their diets, they will greatly reduce this burden. The government and international bodies worldwide should try and educate people so that they can understand that their eating habits have consequences. Policies should be put in place that will generate essential help to people involved in agricultural sectors so that increase of fresh healthy foods could be grown. This will greatly improve people's health and further reduce non-communicable disease in all regions of the world."

Colon cancer has been found to be the second largest leading cause of cancer death in the US and other western countries as opposed to Africa. To test the reason for this disparity, a study was carried out by Professor Jeremy Nicholson and his team of International scientists from the Imperial College London and the University of Pittsburg. They gathered two groups i.e. 20 African Americans from Pittsburgh and 20 rural South Africans from KwaZulu Natal.

The study required the two groups to swap diets under controlled conditions for 14 days. Each participant was a given a colonoscopy examination before the swap was started and after the swap was finished. They also measured biological markers that indicate colon cancer risk and studied the samples of bacteria taken from their colons.

The colonoscopy examination revealed that almost half of the African American participants had abnormal growths in the colon that can progress to cancer, while the Africans did not. After the 14-day swap of diets between the two groups, the African American group had less colon inflammation and there was a drop in multiple risk factors for cancer. On the other hand, the rural African group's cancer risk increased after only 14 days.

Professor Jeremy Nicholson concluded that people can greatly lower their risk of colon cancer by eating foods containing high fiber. He continued to say that it was quite shocking to see that, just after 2 weeks, the risk of cancer in the African participants had dramatically increased than before they started the study, leaving people to raise concerns about the progressive westernization of the African countries today, especially the diet.

Unfortunately, African countries have shifted to western diets over the years. Incidences of cancer are increasing in countries like Kenya and South Africa where the urban populace and the upper class and growing middle class have joined the fast food bandwagon, causing them to change food choices due to the increased wealth of people living in these countries. The growing cases of urban cancer in Africa proves the direct correlation between cancer and diet.

These African countries can better afford the otherwise expensive fast foods that are promoted and sold by the rich countries and their global fast food outlets. However, these foods lead to a greater risk of developing cancer. It has wrongly been sold by the rich countries that progress or development means unhealthy processed foods.

Processed foods have been found to be carcinogenic since they contain chemicals and additives that help the growth of cancer tumors in the human body. Foods like red processed meat, processed foods, and sugary drinks are some of the foods and drinks these countries have adopted as part of their daily diet.

Favorably, not all areas in these developing countries have increased their intake of processed foods. Rural areas have stuck to their diet of eating healthy foods that are a source of fighting cancer and gives them the required nutrients their body needs.

These developing countries should return to consuming healthy foods like fruits, vegetables, and whole grains if they are to have a fighting chance against cancer. They can greatly reduce the rate at which cancer incidences are growing. Another lifestyle change that they could revert to is the reduction of smoking rates which can increase the chance of getting lung cancer.

There are three things that people should know about eating to beat cancer:

- **A good diet increases your chances of surviving cancer and it can also prevent cancer from returning**.
- You should **eat plenty of vegetables and fruits since they have bioactive natural compounds to fight off cancer cells**. Try eating low carbs, low sugar, high-fat natural foods and lots of fibers if you are to have a fighting chance.
- Lastly, **consume good quality supplements that** are all natural. Natural compounds like curcumin, piperine, vitamin E and A, EGCG from green tea and resveratrol could greatly help to stop cancer tumor cells growth.

Once you have these three main tips in mind, your risk of developing cancer will reduce considerably.

Rich Countries Eat Poorer

A lot of research has been done on eating habits in rich countries and the studies have always concluded that processed foods lead to a higher risk of cancer developing. These foods account for the reason why most there is a growing number of people being diagnosed with cancer every year.

Foods that have chemicals in them like refined sugars and artificial sweeteners increase the risk of cancer development. These foods are rich in calories, sodium, and sugar, all of which are harmful to the human body when consumed excessively in the processed form.

Such foods can also lead to obesity which presents another assortment of health problems. Obesity is caused by an unhealthy diet and infrequent exercise. An unhealthy body raises cancer risk.

Processed foods account for 60 percent of foods in the average American diet and 50 percent in the Canadian and United Kingdom diet. This means that half of the citizens in these rich countries' diet consist of consuming unhealthy foods. This is quite dangerous and confirms why these countries record more cancer diagnosis each year than other countries in the world.

Chapter Summary

The risk of developing cancer is greatly influenced by where a person lives and the specific environmental factors that affect their diet. People living in developed countries have a high risk of developing cancer than people living in developing countries.

This is because people living in developed countries consume a diet of more processed unhealthy foods, which is sold as and is considered to be more delicious and 'developed' as opposed to consuming natural foods, which have the most nutrients and will fight cancer and other diseases.

Chapter 4

It's The Food

So, what exactly is the connection between cancer and diet?

Cancer has been linked to diet because food has the power to prevent or contribute to certain types of cancer. Diet is something that you can control and change, and it is more favorable for you to change your diet than to risk developing cancer.

Foods That Increase Cancer Risk

Certain dietary habits have greatly influenced the development of cancer. The following is a look at dietary aspects that commonly lead to the development of cancer:

Characteristics of processed cancer-causing foods

Processed foods have various cancer-causing characteristics. One of these characteristics is that **these foods measure highest in added sugars and salt, as wells as saturated fats.** They **contain lower fiber and vitamins in their make-up** which makes them more cancerous to the human body.

Another characteristic of these processed foods is that **because of packaging, the foods may become contaminated with potentially harmful substances** that could greatly increase the rate of cancer risk. These packages have additional chemicals like wraps that contain plastic cancer chemicals additives that are quite harmful.

The foods themselves **can also contain harmful additives**, which, though approved for use by the U.S. Food and Drug Administration (FDA), have been found to cause cancer in animal and cell studies. They include such additives like processed meat additive, sodium nitrate, and the white food pigment titanium dioxide.

Some of the unhealthy processed foods consumed regularly are; fish nuggets, packaged sweet and savory snacks, meat products that have been reconstituted with the aid of nitrites or other salt preservatives, packaged bread, foods made mostly from sugars, oils, and fats.

These foods contain harmful substances from industrial processing like flavoring agents, color, humectants, emulsifiers and artificial sweeteners. These harmful substances are usually added to imitate sensorial properties or disguise undesirable qualities.

Therefore, unprocessed foods have a very big impact on the control and prevention of cancer. Quite sadly, despite all the technological advances and the high standard of living, the majority of people in developed countries do not eat healthy foods.

Salty foods: These are foods which contain a very high measure of sodium. It is estimated that 9.5 percent of cancer deaths are related to consuming foods containing high salt intake.

Another excessively common food in developed countries is **processed red meat**. From pork, beef to mutton, all these meats undergo an industrial processing where certain chemicals are added to them to preserve their shelf lives and also to make them tastier by adding artificial flavors.

Processed meat is meat that has been passed through the process of being smoked, fermented or salted, and nitrites added to enhance flavor. Eating 50 grams of processed meat every day is associated with an increase in colorectal cancer risk. Red meat is also included in this fact since red meat also contains iron.

Sugary sweets and sodas are pure chemicals with lots of unhealthy sugars. Not one soda that is produced is made up of any fruits or is fruit based. They account for almost 80 percent of cancer deaths in rich countries because these are the compounds that feed cancer cells up to a point where they can replicate themselves in different parts of the body.

Glycemic index can be described as a measure of how fast carbohydrates turn into sugar in the blood. Consumption of foods with a GI of 70 or above is associated with 88 percent of developing prostate cancer. These foods include things like sugar-sweetened drinks, fruit juices, processed foods like pizza, etc. It is more beneficial to eat low GI foods like legumes so as to minimize the risk of developing prostate cancer.

Further, the people in rich countries do not consume as many fruits as they should. They would rather have an artificially flavored drink than eat fruits. The minimal consumption of fresh fruits lowers immunity and causes them not to have a fighting chance against cancer.

Foods That Lower Cancer Risk

Now that we have touched on the foods that increase the risk of developing cancer, which foods are best at reducing cancer risk?

Antioxidants are known to prevent cancer because they help in neutralizing radicals that damage cells. People should aim for a diet that includes a variety of high oxidants unlike targeting individual oxidants for best results such as those found in tablets and pills.

Calcium is another dietary supplement that helps to lower the risk for cancer in the body. Calcium binds to bile acids and fatty acids in gastrointestinal to protect cells from damaging stomach acids. Since too much of something is poison, consuming too much calcium per day is linked to having a higher risk of developing prostate cancer. People should try to consume up to a maximum of 1000mg per day.

Fruits and vegetables are rich in antioxidants. Nuts, beans, whole grains and healthy fats are also some of the foods that you should consume if you are to have a chance at surviving a cancer diagnosis. Try as much as possible to limit unhealthy fats, fried foods, processed meats, sugars, and refined carbs since they can counteract the effects of these antioxidants. Vegetables are very important for fighting cancer because of the high fiber content and they also contain beneficial vitamins that would be a great help in the body if consumed.

Some of the vegetables available with high antioxidants are carrots, brussels sprouts, and squash. These are known to reduce the risk of developing lung cancer, mouth cancer, pharynx cancer and larynx cancer. Other vegetables like non-starchy vegetables (broccoli, spinach and, beans) help with protection from stomach cancer and esophageal cancer.

Oranges, berries, peas, bell peppers, and dark leafy greens are rich in vitamin C, which is handy when it comes to protecting against esophageal cancer. Tomatoes, guava, and watermelon are foods high in lycopene which is a supplement responsible for helping the body by protecting it from prostate cancer.

If people incorporated fruits and vegetables into their diet their cancer risk would decrease exponentially. Most people fall short of the daily recommended minimum serving of fruits and vegetables and that is why their risk of cancer development is high. You should try to focus on adding wholemeal foods to your diet and try to consume natural foods rather than processed foods.

Dietary Weight Control

Weight gain is a very crucial factor when it is linked to cancer. When you control your weight through dietary modification, you are more protected from the risk of developing cancer than when you just ignore it. People with a higher body mass index risk developing some common cancers like colon cancer, gallbladder, kidney and liver cancer. This is because body fat produces hormones and inflammatory proteins the can greatly promote the growth of the tumor cells.

CHAPTER SUMMARY

Lifestyle plays a greater role in controlling cancer than any other factor. A combination of a good diet and other healthy habits can greatly lower the risk of developing cancer. Lifestyle changes like quitting smoking, stopping alcohol consumption, and weight control management are some of the ways that can be adopted if you are to have a good chance of controlling cancer.

Diet has a direct link to the risk of developing cancer. Depending on how one chooses to eat, whether the 'Western' diet or one that is natural and healthy, the risk of developing cancer can increase or decrease respectively.

Foods rich in natural nutrients and fiber should be consumed more to better develop immunity and increase survival chances against cancer. Diet and lifestyle go hand in hand and if one can adopt a healthy diet and lifestyle, then cancer will be controlled.

Make the change today because regardless of your location, you can opt for a more natural, healthier diet.

Chapter 5

The Diet That Causes Cancer

Diet is a crucial factor in the increasing incidences of cancer and prevention of cancer. Food has been responsible for more than 30 percent of cancer cases all over the world, making it the highest cause of cancer development.

Certain foods have such high carcinogens thus triggering and escalating the spread of cancer cells in the body. An alteration of diet can give the body a high chance to fight off cancer cells, more than any other factors including treatment.

Here, we are going to explore some common foods that cause cancer and the changes that people should adopt if they want to prevent or survive it.

Foods That Cause Cancer

As we have already established, food plays a very big role when it comes to preventing, controlling, and curing cancer in the human body. Many of the foods today contain a lot of carcinogens from fertilizers that are used in growing food crops and from the manufacturing process of industrialized foods (processed foods).

More recently, the science of genetically modified foods has been signaled as a possible contributor to cancer because of the alteration of animal or plant genetic makeup occasioned in the process.

Genetically Modified Foods

Genetically modified foods (GMOs) involves altering the DNA constitution of plants and animals that are used as food. GMOs are plants and animals created by inserting genes from one species to another. It can also be called 'splicing' (a term in genetic engineering) and it is often done in a lab.

Splicing is done so that it can enhance certain desired traits in the plant or animal, for example, to make the plant more resistant to pesticides, killer weeds or disease, to harden plants to survive winter and droughts or improve animal nutritional content.

GMO foods have been linked to the development of cancer in the long term since cancer is an illness that comes later in life. People should try and know which crops have been genetically modified so that they can understand how well to reduce the risk of developing cancer by limiting or avoiding their consumption.

Crops like soybeans, corn, cotton (used in the production of oil), canola (for making oil), squash, zucchini, and papaya are all great examples of foods that have been genetically modified.

Organic plant foods grown organically from non-GMO seeds of plants are the best. Meat from grass-fed animals should be consumed rather than animals that have been fed with GMO animal feeds like modified corn or alfalfa for cows. One should also avoid ingredients like corn syrup and lecithin because these ingredients pass through major modification to become finished products.

Non-organic Produce

Non-organic foods are those that have been exposed to harmful pesticides and chemicals. Pesticides and chemicals are used to control and kill insects, weeds and fungal pests that might damage the crops. These non-organic foods are also treated with a variety of growth-enhancing chemicals that give them a bigger structure and a clean appearance when compared to organic food.

You should realize that you are what you eat. The health risk associated with pesticides is quite immense and negating the risk can only be good for your health. Although organic foods are quite expensive, they are worth every penny when it comes to eating healthy and keeping your family safe from developing diseases like cancer. If you have a piece of land that you can turn into a garden, you should try as much as possible to grow your own food. If you are buying from a grocery, you should purchase conventional produce and stay away from foods that contain chemicals.

Canned Foods

Canned foods are those stored in cans and sold in supermarkets and other stores. They contain bisphenol which is a man-made industrial chemical that is used to make hard, clear plastic used for food and drink packaging, microwave ovenware, storage containers, and water and milk bottles.

It is also used in making epoxy resins which lines the cans of canned food like baked beans, soup, tomatoes and cans of fizzy and alcoholic drinks. This chemical has been linked to the development of breast cancer and prostate cancer. Consumers should opt for foods packaged in glass and other non-can materials when possible.

<u>Refined Sugar</u>

Refined sugar is a sugar high in fructose corn syrup. Refines sugar is the major source of insulin spikes and it greatly increases the risk of developing cancer cells. Refined sugar is white sugar from sugar canes and sugar beets which pass through the process of extraction to get the sugar. It is a combination of glucose and fructose which makes up sucrose.

Today, more refined sugar is eaten than ever before, especially compared to the times of our parents and grandparents decades ago. This has increased the rate of obesity in adults and children and obesity has been linked to certain cancers like breast cancer, prostate cancer, uterine cancer, colorectal and pancreatic cancer.

You should avoid refined/white sugar and go for brown sugar or no sugar at all. When you start to control your sugar intake, the resulting healthier immune system will help the body fight off cancer cells in the body and act as a preventive measure against cancer.

White Flour

White flour can be described as refined flour where all nutritional value in the flour including natural fiber is removed and it is then bleached with chlorine gas so that it can look appealing to consumers. White flour has the ability to spike your insulin levels without it really providing nutritional fuel to your body.

Due to the lack of nutritional content in white flour, the insulin that is produced, due to this flour, only further makes the body receptive to cancer. Cancer has been found to flourish in a body that is producing a lot of sugar and white flour only encourages the body to produce insulin which helps breaks down the fats in the body making glucose to feed cancer cells.

White flour is highly unhealthy and you should opt for whole grain wheat instead.

Microwave Popcorn

Microwave popcorn can be described as popcorn that pops while it is still inside the chemically lined package bag that is put inside the microwave for heating. It is closely linked to lung cancer since the bag and the oil are highly toxic to the body.

Diacetyl is a chemical that is added to these popcorns to give them an artificial butter flavor and it has been linked to a rare type of lung cancer also known as "popcorn worker's lung." The only way to cure this type of cancer is to get a lung transplant because it damages the lung beyond repair.

Try to let the popcorn cool down before you pop the bag. Diacetyl is more deadly if you inhale the hot vapor directly from the bag while hot. Try and get organic popcorns which you can pop over a stove using a covered pan with a little oil. This way, you can avoid consuming the genetically modified ingredients in these popcorn bags.

Potato Chips

Potato chips are a snack prepared by deep frying slices of potatoes in hot oil at high temperatures. Cooking starchy foods like potatoes at high temperatures can lead to cancer.

Acrylamide is a by-product chemical that is produced after exposing these starchy foods to very high temperatures. This chemical is rapidly absorbed and distributed all over the body which then increases the risk of damaging DNA and causes genetic mutations.

Another carcinogenic compound that is produced during the cooking of potato chips is polycyclic aromatic hydrocarbons. This is a compound that is found in the air as smoke from the grill, oven or stove while cooking rises. Once one inhales this carbon, it enters the body and causes major complications.

Heterocyclic amines are also a by-product of cooking potato chips at high temperatures. If they are overcooked, they produce this toxic compound. Once consumed, the risk of developing cancer increases.

It is advised that you avoid potato chips because their effects are more severe than in any other food group.

Red Meat

Heterocyclic aromatic amines is a compound that is produced from grilling red meat. It is carcinogenic and it is directly linked to cancer development. Consumption of meat has also been linked to several cancer cases because the chemicals formed during the digestion of meat have been found to damage cells lining the bowels.

The fat content in meat is also a factor to consider when linking meat to cancer because meat does not have protective properties like in fruits, vegetables, and whole grain cereals.

You should reduce weekly meat intake. Around 455 grams of meat per week is recommended if you desire to reduce your risk of developing cancer.

Processed Meat

Processed meat is meat that has been treated to preserve or flavor it. Meats like hot dogs, ham, sausages, and other deli meats are some of the few examples of processed meats. The processing methods include salting, curing, fermenting, and smoking.

Processed meat has been linked to the development of cancer regardless of the quantity of processed meat one takes. The methods of processing these meats are known to contain carcinogens that are radioactive and are commonly known to interfere with the consumer's DNA, leaving one at a high risk of developing cancer.

There is no recommended quantity of processed meat that one should consume because it is all unsafe as far as cancer is concerned.

<u>Farmed Raised Fish</u>

Commercial farming has become very widespread today. It involves raising a large number of fish (e.g. salmon) in a crowded environment compared to fish found in the wild. Fish farming involves the use of antibiotics, pesticides, and other carcinogenic chemicals to control bacteria and viruses in the pond water.

Farmed fish are known to produce omega 6 fatty acids which can cause inflammations in the human body including an increase in the development of cancer cells in the body. The use of antibiotic in these fish can make the human body resistant to antibiotics which you may need when sick.

You should always seek out wild fish when possible since these fish are rich in omega 3 fatty acids and other natural nutrients devoid of contamination as compared to farmed fish. Avoid farmed fish which are highly toxic.

Hydrogenated Oils

These are vegetable oils whose structure has been changed through a process of hydrogenation to increase the shelf life. This process changes the taste and smell and elevates its saturated fats content while decreasing unsaturated fat.

Hydrogenated oils have unhealthy omega 6 fatty acids and have been known to alter the structure of the cell membrane.

These oils have been linked to the growing incidences of colorectal cancer in the world. They contain a high percentage of cholesterol which is unhealthy. These oils are used to make other human consumables like margarine which is unhealthy. To fight cancer, avoid hydrogenated oils.

Anything Labeled Diet

Diet labeled foods have grown in popularity because they are touted as the alternative to the unhealthy processed foods but are they really safe and healthy?

Well, as much as diet labeled items do not contain refined sugars, they contain artificial sugars which are also not safe when speaking about cancer. Artificial sweeteners create changes in your body and brain. Therefore, these are hardly safe.

Drinks That Cause Cancer

In cancer research circles, sugar is regarded as the fuel which feeds cancer cells and a chemical which damages the human body to an extent that it forms cancer cells. Drinks like sodas and carbonated drinks have so much sugar that they render the body unhealthy and inflamed, leaving it susceptible to diseases such as cancer.

However, there are other drinks that you should avoid.

Alcoholic Beverages

Alcohol is a term used to describe an agent called ethanol which is found in beer, wine, and liquors. It is also found in medicine, mouthwashes, household products and essential oils. It is usually produced as a result of fermentation of sugars and starches by yeast.

Alcohol consumption has been linked to the development of different types of cancers in the human body. Some of these cancers are head and neck cancer, esophageal cancer, liver cancer, breast cancer, and stomach cancer. The risk of cancer actually doubles when someone indulges in alcoholic beverages than when he or she does not indulge.

There are a variety of carcinogenic contaminants in alcoholic beverages introduced during the fermentation process such as hydrocarbons. Sugars contained in alcoholic beverages have also been known to be a big contributor to the development of cancer cells.

Little to no alcohol should be the way if you are to steer clear of cancer.

Soda and Carbonated Beverages

Soda is one of the most discussed beverages because of its unhealthy qualities. It is filled with fructose, dyes, and a lot more chemicals making it very bad for your health. Soda does not have any nutritional value and only adds to your calorie intake.

Soda and carbonated water contain CO_2 as the active ingredient. The CO_2 is pressurized into the water and the soda creating an effervescent bubble. Someone who has been diagnosed with cancer should be very aware that these carbonated drinks only add salt to their already injured body.

Carbonated drinks also contain added sugars which have been proved to be the fuel that feeds cancer cells. Sugars occurring naturally like in fruits should be encouraged because they act as a primary energy source in the body compared to these artificial sugars in processed drinks and foods.

Artificial Sweeteners

Artificial sweeteners are basically your normal sugar substitutes and are much sweeter than sucrose in much smaller quantities.

Early research of artificial sweeteners showed that combining cyclamate with saccharin caused bladder cancer in laboratory animals thus the association with cancer. However, subsequent carcinogenicity studies have not yielded clear evidence or proof of cancer development in human beings.

Despite the inconclusive research, artificial sweeteners contribute to the exacerbation and development of other health problems like obesity and kidney problems and are highly suspected to be a catalyst for cancer like processed sugar.

Studies by Brian Hoffmann, assistant professor in the Department of Biomedical Engineering at the Medical College of Wisconsin and Marquette University, in lab animals show that artificial sweeteners cause metabolic disorders by altering the activity of certain genes responsible for breaking down macromolecules such as fats and proteins.

Chapter Summary

Cancer-causing foods are foods that increase the risk of developing cancer in the human body. These foods contain carcinogenic compounds that make the body very susceptible to developing cancer cells or accelerate the growth of cancer cells.

When it comes to a cancer-fighting diet, the only way to go is organic foods. Natural foods must dominate your plate with every meal you eat. Realistically, it is virtually impossible to completely avoid the unhealthy foods but there is a way around it.

Instead of drinking soda three times a day with every meal you eat, you can choose to drink it once a week. Rather than make fast food your staple, you can choose to cook and eat better meals. It all boils down to a choice.

Diet plays a major role in the prevention, control, and cure of cancer. Make the choice to avoid the diet that causes cancer. Eat natural, eat healthily.

About the Author

Sienna Silverton is passionate about fitness and health education. Sienna enjoys educating people on natural remedies to improve mental and physical health. Besides engaging in gym activities like weight training and spinning in her spare time, she also enjoying salsa dancing with friends on weekends and binge-watching on Netflix.

www.ingramcontent.com/pod-product-compliance
Lightning Source LLC
Chambersburg PA
CBHW071432220526
45469CB00004B/1501